through

the EYES

of *dementia*

Through *the* Eyes *of* Dementia

A Pocket Guide to Caregiving

Johnna Lowther

This book is intended as a guide and is meant for educational and informational purposes only. This book is not a substitute for seeking diagnosis, treatment, or care advice from a physician or other qualified healthcare provider.

The individual experiences recounted in this book are true. However, some names and details may have been changed for privacy.

For information, address JoJo Studio Press.

ISBN: 1499731485
ISBN-13: 978-1499731484

1. Dementia--Patients. 2. Alzheimer's Disease--Patients. 3. Family--
   Caregivers. 4. Dementia--Brain disorder. 5. Consulting--Health--
   Diseases--Caregiving.

Cover art: Frances LaSala
Cover design: Laura Beers
Author photograph back cover: Peggy Stanley

Published by
JoJo Studio Press
Kansas City, MO
Email: jojostudiopress@gmail.com
facebook.com/ThroughTheEyesOfDementia

DEDICATION

*To those who fight this disease every single day and
the families that have changed my life forever.*

ACKNOWLEDGMENTS

I am in absolute gratitude to the friends and professionals whom I consulted for editing, design and format. It is their collaboration that made this book possible. A very special thanks to: Lori Wilber, Laura Beers, Carol Babcock and Jenay Morrisey for their individual touches and professional advice that helped make the beauty of this book shine through.

Thank you.

ABOUT THE ARTWORK

The image on the cover of this book was beautifully created by Frances, one of my friends with dementia. I am thankful to her family for allowing me to honor her life and speak of the dynamic person I believe her to be. In my mind, she was the epitome of an Italian grandma. You know the type: tiny - but a mighty force to be dealt with. But oh when she loved, she showered it upon you like you were the only one in the room! She'd kiss your cheeks and squeeze them, as she would say, *"You are just so precious! Just precious! You are a doll you know that? And don't let anyone tell you different!"* And you could feel every exclamation point at the end of her sentences. I envy the vitality for life that seems to be present in the culture of Italian women. They never stop moving; like a bottomless pot of pasta e fagioli, they just keep nourishing the family that surrounds them. You can see in her brushstrokes the force of energy behind the paint as it moves across the paper.

The positive effect that artistic outlets and creative therapies offer those battling Alzheimer's and other dementias continues to blow my mind. Research has discovered that the non-analytical sections of the brain are the last to be altered by the disease. By tapping into the creative side of the brain you can access a powerful tool for communication. Offering various opportunities to engage and interact with persons is vitally important to daily living in the world of dementia.

"Music and art stimulate the brain in areas that Alzheimer's cannot touch, bypassing the debilitating disease and often providing relief. Engaging in activities like arts and crafts, music, meditation, home repair and reading stimulate the mind, reduces the effect of stress-related diseases, and slows cognitive decline."
- www.CreativeAging.org

One of the most inspiring programs I've had the honor of developing was an intergenerational art project. This project began as an opportunity to connect seniors and youth through creative exchange and unite generations in collaboration. Ranging in age from four to ninety-four, some grandparents partnering with their great grand-children, they participated in a group project centered on the common bond of expression through art. I invited families, community youth, and children's groups to join and together, create a piece of work. There were retired art instructors in the group, soccer players, social studies majors, science and math students, and many who actively used art and creative writing as a personal form of expression. Learning, growing, visiting old memories and making new ones were all some of the side goals of this project. The real success was seen in the rich collab-oration between generations and the expressions of joy that were shared in the moment. Observing and facil-itating these interactions have become moments in time that now make up some of the most precious images burned in my brain.

"It's not what you look at that matters.
It's what you see." - *Henry David Thoreau*

contents

ONE
Being Vulnerable   25

TWO
Understanding the Disease   33

THREE
Inclusion Therapy   39

FOUR
Know Their Needs   49

FIVE
Communicate Effectively   57

SIX
Offer Acceptance   69

SEVEN
Renew a Sense of Control   75

EIGHT
Don't Argue   83

NINE
Redirection and Distraction   89

TEN
Laugh It Off   97

ELEVEN
Remain Calm   101

TWELVE
Be Consistent   107

THIRTEEN
Using Therapeutic Outlets   111

FOURTEEN
Give Love   127

Johnna Lowther stands apart among professionals working in the field of aging. It is evident that she loves what she does and has a special kind of empathy and enthusiasm for caring. She wears creativity as a style; a significant way of working with people. This flair, mixed with her sensitivity is able to attract people into authentic exchange. When Johnna is interacting with persons who are cognitively impaired, she is mindful and present; positive and energetic. She validates each person's contribution, acknowledging worth and dignity, and connects to the person beneath the disease. This warm energy is vital to working with persons with dementia.

I have worked in the field of aging for over twenty years, as an educator in social gerontology, a drama therapist and a social services provider. Over the past few years, I have had many opportunities to watch Johnna's daily encounters with residents of a memory care center, in a variety of settings and diverse circumstances. Witnessing her working, I see tenderness and unhurried calm. She is able to diffuse and disarm situations that might otherwise escalate with confusion. She uplifts each person and situation with a quiet confidence and brings a lightheartedness that is simultaneously sincere.

I believe that Johnna's greatest expertise comes from her strong intuition. She is in-tune with the needs of dementia and establishes relationships built on a true sense of trust. While it is debatable whether or not intuition is teachable, she inspires the desire to build a framework of intuition; to trust it; and hone skills that build meaningful connections with persons who have Alzheimer's or dementia. These skills compliment her professionalism and confirm that Johnna knows exactly what she is doing. My collaborations with her have changed the way I now work with persons who have dementia for she has elevated caregiving to an art form.

With so many books about the how-tos of caregiving and activities meant to engage loved ones; why do I put weight in what Johnna Lowther has to say? Why listen to her ideas? I believe we listen because she has a new voice and a fresh perspective. I've seen her interventions, and they work. I know that she writes from a place of real knowledge and hands on experience. What she has to say is grounded in rich and meaningful encounters.

At a glance, Johnna's techniques may seem simple and easy. That's just it! It is the ease that sets her apart and makes her contributions to this field so valuable. My respect and appreciation for Johnna's work is because at the heart of her approach, is a purposeful simplicity. I hope that *Through the Eyes of Dementia* will bring more meaning to your interactions in caregiving and touch your heart, as she has done for so many others.

-Deb Campbell
Drama Therapist, M.S. Gerontology
Executive Director, Kansas City Senior Theatre

My Story

Alzheimer's disease and dementia is an illness especially hard on families. I know because I've experienced it in my family. You essentially experience loss on a continual basis. It's never easy to lose a loved one. But watching them die a new death through each stage they progress is very difficult. Working in the field of dementia care, I see individuals at many stages of the disease process. The early stages seem especially tough on the patient because they are more aware of their personal loss. I think it's easier somewhere in the middle stages, when most seem "deliriously happy". But no matter how you look at it, from the perspective of the person battling the disease or that of the family member, it's a tough road. Yet, through my work, I see the beauty of the moments in between. I get to be a bridge for both sides, leading them out of sadness and into a moment of joy, even if that moment may only last minutes. That's why I love my job. I consider it a rare gift to observe people experiencing joy, and the fact that I get to join them there is very gratifying.

Years of facilitating support groups and countless conversations with residents and families have prompted me to write on the topic of caregiving; and so began my collection of writings. Being a caregiver for a person with dementia requires some extra special sleuthing skills sometimes. We try to understand and interpret the words that make no sense or find meaning in the strange actions of someone with dementia, who is desperately trying to communicate. It's not always easy. In fact, it can be very hard, and will try the patience of the most kind and loving human beings on the planet.

As I've listened to the words of family members experiencing changes in the relationship with their loved one and not knowing what to do, I realized that so much of what I happen "to know" by working in this field, is not always known to the families and caregivers dealing with this disease. That's exactly where I want to make a difference. I want this book to be a resource that helps make this process less painful for everyone involved. I also want to give the person with dementia a public voice; something that says:

*"I'm still here...
and this is hard for me too."*

Because it is, hard for them. I want to validate family members feelings and offer solutions to encourage a successful relationship with the new person their loved one is now becoming. I hope that by practicing these techniques, your caregiving experience can be more peaceful and I hope that you will feel less lonely. If I am able to make one heart a little less heavy and one-step a little bit lighter in this journey, then I will feel I have succeeded.

There are countless resources and excellent writers on this topic; with many more on the way as the discussion of Alzheimer's disease and dementia continues to become more prevalent in our society. I have designed this book to be a quick and easy guide for families and caregivers. I see you. I hear you. I am one of you. I feel your pain as you are working tirelessly to meet the needs of those living a life with dementia. This is now your "pocket guide". You can throw it in your purse or bag and pull it out in a waiting room; at the doctor's office; traveling on a plane; taking a break at your local coffee shop or in the comfort of your own home. If you learn one thing from it, I hope you share it with someone else. May it be of help and comfort as you are learning to live with dementia in your life.

one

Being Vulnerable

*Vulnerability brings empathy and with
empathy comes understanding.*

Life should be about fulfillment. Not money, not jobs, not possessions, not whether we're sick or well. But about finding fulfillment wherever we are. That is what my occupation is all about. At least, those are my personal convictions surrounding the job that I do. I work with persons affected by Alzheimer's disease and other dementias. Basically, I help make confused people happy or end my day trying to. These people surprise me in a very deep and affectionate form and there is a rich, personal joy in those moments. There are no predetermined thoughts or expectations and that's what I love about sharing their life. It's like a new day every day because it's not boxed in with agendas. It's totally fresh.

I fell into this line of work rather by accident. As a young college student, I answered an ad for a part-time job at a local nursing home, leading activities with the residents there. Upon interviewing, they explained I would be working on their secured care unit for residents with Alzheimer's and dementia. This job changed my life. I had a wonderful co-worker named Dela, to whom I credit mentoring within me a calm, sincere and loving approach. She never raised her voice, always gave her complete attention and lovingly caressed the hands and hearts of those residents. She made them feel like there was nothing else more important than them.

It was a fulfilling experience for both her and the person she was sharing these moments with, and I soaked that up like a sponge. She opened her heart and created a safe haven where those with dementia could reveal themselves. It was the ultimate foundation for trust. But it wasn't just Dela who taught me. The residents I worked with and subsequent relationships I formed forever impacted the words, tone and energy I now project in my work.

The life of a person with dementia is very much in the moment. As control over their mind begins to fade, their emotions are less inhibited and they become quite sensitive to non-verbal interaction. I firmly believe that the energy you emit *directly* reflects in those surrounding you and vice versa. This is why it's important that we, as caregivers, take our attitude and negative factors that get thrown at us on a daily basis and somehow find a way to reflect this energy in a positive dynamic. You can do this by letting go of expectations and the desire to control what's happening. Dementia gives its victim no choice in the matter; it demands control. No one has control over this disease. I have learned through the years that the more I give and share of myself, the more fulfilling my caregiving experience has been. Relinquishing control opens the door to vulnerability. But it also offers an opportunity for reflection, intimacy and growth. Vulnerability brings empathy; and with empathy comes understanding.

It is important to remember that those battling dementia no longer have control over their own thoughts, emotions and therefore actions. When you become frustrated in dealing with this, realize that it's equally and even more frustrating for the person with the disease. How demeaning would it feel if you had no choice over what's happening to you? Making decisions are how we learn to both express and experience enjoyment in our lives, and the majority of healthy individuals live their life doing this. Imagine how it would feel if that ability were taken away from you. Empathizing with this feeling is why I am so passionate about working in this field. I want us to care for these individuals in a way that brings joy to their every day, waking moments.

It may seem as though your loved one is a completely different person. You're right. They have lost control of their body, their brain and their life. Your loss is also their loss. Cry with them. Hug them. Hold them. Be angry together, but not at each other. Embrace the common bond between your feelings. What's happening is not your fault. It's not their fault. It's the uncontrollable factor of Alzheimer's disease and dementia causing this loss.

I remain humbled by what a person battling dementia can teach me. I think back to a particular man I worked with in mid-to-late stages of Alzheimer's disease. His whole life he had been an integral part of his church choir and was a lead cantor for the congregation. During this particular visit, we were using rhythm therapy, playing specific patterns on hand drums and taking turns leading, following and repeating. I remember how as the rhythm shifted, his hands and body began to move to a place that was not in that present moment. It was as though he had traveled to a space beyond his mind, that his body remembered all too well and I was a mere observer of the journey. In less than sixty seconds he taught me an eternal lesson:

> *"The spirit never forgets and it knows*
> *the origin from which it comes."*

The ability for a person with dementia to express the knowledge and memories within becomes more and more inhibited as the disease progresses. But if, and when, the mind retains something it can turn and pass on, therein lies the gift.

The purity of an Alzheimer's disease patient; this is what moves me. I want you, as a friend, a loved one, a caregiver or even a stranger, to know this person within. I want you to read between the lines, see beyond the words that make no sense and embrace this person for all that they were, currently are and also who they are now becoming. Yes, it is painful; but the sweet moments that come out of this vulnerability can also bring a healing otherwise lost. Open up and give this new person a place in your life. This gift will never fade.

two

Understanding the Disease

*If we are to be better caregivers, we must
continually learn, as much as we can about
Alzheimer's disease and dementia.*

Dementia is cognitive loss due to injury or insult to the brain. Many different things can cause dementia: certain forms of cancer, stroke, head trauma, or Parkinson's disease, to name a few. The distinction of Alzheimer's disease is the fact that it is an irreversible form of dementia. An article by Cheryl Arnella, *"Alzheimer's Disease (and other Brain Diseases) and Hospice Care"* references Alzheimer's Disease as: "a progressive, neurodegenerative disease characterized by loss of function and death of nerve cells in several areas of the brain. This leads to loss of cognitive function such as memory and language." Put simply, Alzheimer's is a permanent digression of the brain. In the end, it will become compromised to the point of death. For those battling the disease, this sad reality only heightens the importance of living in the present moment. Each moment in the life of an Alzheimer's patient is a precious breath, for who knows how long that moment and level of cognition or function will last.

In "Alzheimer's Disease: The Dignity Within" by Patricia Callone, et al., it states that Alzheimer's disease is the fourth leading cause of death after heart disease, cancer and stroke. This disease is rapidly growing. Progression of the disease moves at a different rate for each individual. I have worked in senior living centers since 2001, and have observed residents who live in various levels, or stages, of the disease for many years and yet others who experience very rapid changes. I lost a grandfather who maintained in the very early stages for at least ten years and then moved through moderate and severe stages in less than a year and a half, finally taking his life.

It's painful and difficult for both the caregivers and the person experiencing the symptoms of this disease. The subsequent loss experienced by both individuals is hard to understand unless you've been there. But if we are to be better in this field of caregiving, we must continue to learn and understand as much as we can about Alzheimer's disease and dementia.

The Alzheimer's Association recognizes 7 stages of the disease:

Stage 1: No impairment
Stage 2: Very mild decline
Stage 3: Mild decline
Stage 4: Moderate decline
Stage 5: Moderately severe decline
Stage 6: Severe decline
Stage 7: Very severe decline

The Alzheimer's Association is an amazing support system for families, patients and caregivers; and they have countless resources to guide you through this process. I personally have attended many of their professional education sessions and credit them with my better understanding of appropriate caregiving. To visit their website or find a local chapter in your area, go to: www.alz.org. I will again reference "Alzheimer's Disease: The Dignity Within" by Patricia R. Callone, et al. as they do an excellent job condensing the stages of this disease into three categories: early-to-mild, moderate and severe.

- **Early-to-mild stage**: the person has trouble remembering but can often describe his or her problems clearly and can continue to do most of the things they have always done.

- **Moderate stage**: the brain deteriorates more and personality changes can occur.

- **Severe stage**: the individual becomes relatively nonfunctional and is often confined to bed.

Alzheimer's disease strategically moves through the brain, literally eating the tissue as it goes. There are many explanations and descriptions to offer, which can mean different things to each of us dealing with this diagnosis. To be a successful caregiver, you must be prepared for where this disease is going to take both you, your family and your loved one, and it won't always be easy. There will be moments of pain and sorrow. But there will also be moments that shine light upon your soul and bring you great peace. I encourage you to educate and nurture yourself as much as possible. You cannot adequately take care of your loved one if you are not taking care of yourself. I know this, because I've been there. You bring much more strength to the table when you reinforce your foundation. Feed your mind, body and soul and step an inch closer to understanding and believing that it's going to be ok, because it is. You'll get there.

three

Inclusion Therapy

*By being included, persons with dementia
become a living, breathing member of life again.*

I spent much of my childhood struggling to "fit in". I was a tall, thin and gangly child, who ran into walls and doorways for no apparent reason. The social circle of my youth was relatively small and subsequently, my imagination became my best friend. I would make up elaborate tales in my head and entertain myself for hours alone in my room, and was perfectly content doing so. I learned to shrug things off at an early age, which has certainly helped groom my days into adulthood. I realize of course, this experience is probably not unique. Growing up is all about learning how to get comfortable in your own skin. But no matter what your age, it is part of our human existence to interact and systematically learn how things connect and intersect.

our tribe

Most of us spend huge chunks of our lives looking for "our tribe"; people with whom we have similar interests; whom we look to for guidance and collaboration and who in turn will share this thing called "life". In a tribe, when each member contributes, the group as a whole develops strength and sustainability and this sense of belonging stirs within us feelings of joy and contentment.

to feel valued

If there was one thing I could stress about living with dementia, it is this: it is vital that a person battling dementia feel valued, because they experience loss after loss, day after day. Losing a sense of self, family, home, and overall orientation leaves them feeling lost, alone and useless. In the midst of the chaos and confusion in their brain, this person with dementia needs something to remind them that their presence in life matters. Giving them a sense of place, value and personhood in their surrounding environment is the key. Bringing everyone in the community together, as a group, on a regular basis encourages this feeling of purpose and plugs them into a social atmosphere where their communication and involvement matters. By being a member of a tribe, they become an active, living, breathing part of life again.

Years of working in senior living and healthcare have guided me in developing an approach I have termed *inclusion therapy*. The purpose of this technique is to include each person: meaning staff, resident, family, visitor, or even animal, that enters a dementia care setting as a member of the whole.

Inclusion therapy is a form of direct
engagement that puts a high priority on
group activity and social interaction.

The historical culture of elder care in a residential setting had very distinct divisions of labor; each staff member had their individual list of job duties. But this culture is rapidly changing. It is evolving from an institutionalized and departmentalized setting into an environment that puts more power and control in the hands of the client. The new face of senior healthcare focuses on what the industry has termed "person centered care"; which is when care is based on the individual needs and preferences of each resident. In essence, it focuses on the needs of the consumer not the needs of the provider.

Most everyone who has worked in elder care has experienced persons battling memory loss. We hear repetitive questions and attempts of communication that is full of "word salad": forming sentences with words and phrases that don't make sense. We see emotional responses and behavior that, to our perception, do not fit the circumstances. Yet inside the mind of a person with dementia, they recognize our confusion and can get just as frustrated as we are in that moment. Their feelings of self-esteem and value plummet with their inability to communicate. They know something is wrong. I've had residents with Alzheimer's disease tell me:

"I feel so inferior."

As an elder caregiver, having empathy is critical. When you hear how they feel, see what they battle and realize that they did not choose this disease, it changes how you approach your work. A person with dementia *needs* their caregivers to help them feel joy, comfort and peace in their current lives. Understanding the quality of life issues that a person with dementia battles is a continuous learning experience. I've found that by listening and watching, the person with dementia teaches me how to approach, how to speak or act and how to effectively meet their needs. I place a high value on them as a teacher and accept, with great honor, the subsequent knowledge they pass on to me. When I've specifically asked a person in the beginning stages of dementia how living with this disease makes them feel this is their response:

*"It's hard to accept, but I learn
to live with it."*

That could easily be you or me someday, especially at the rate Alzheimer's disease seems to be increasing. My heart goes out to the people of this disease. How frustrating and powerless they must feel!

Specifically in a senior living setting, this is why it's of utmost importance for every staff member to be a part of an overall, engaging environment. When every person is an important member of the whole, it creates a circular program of safety, dignity and validation. Losing your mind is a very scary thing. Have you ever been driving down the road and suddenly realize that you've arrived at a different spot in your journey and don't remember passing certain points? Did it frighten you? Can you imagine doing that every day? How would that make you feel? The goal with inclusion therapy is to create an environment where a person with dementia can thrive and flourish. This is accomplished by building a foundation that is rooted in trust and safety. When caregivers build personal relationships with those they are caring for, they build this trust and make achieving daily tasks more successful. It becomes an active process for both participants and they share the workload, instead of the caregiver doing all the work. If we can learn to empower those with dementia to take action it makes the job of the caregiver, easier.

When we learn to modify our approach, it eliminates the need for interpretation. By implementing inclusion therapy, individuals encourage one another and support each person in participation. Engaging with a group unconsciously motivates the individual to contribute and be a part of the whole as they watch other members interacting. While observing action, one begins to mirror it in their own action because they want to be a part.

As a caregiver of someone with dementia, we must find ways to actively invite and include them in making daily choices.

---

for example:

Let's say it's time for supper. Whether this is in your home, their home or a senior living situation, vocalize the fact that: *"It's time for supper."* Then give the person with dementia a sense of independence by asking: *"Are you ready to eat? I'm hungry. How about you?"* By presenting it in this way, you have included them in the decision making, while gently leading them to respond in acceptance. We must modify *our* actions and approach, instead of the other way around.

hold hope

I reflect back on points in my life where I have felt completely powerless, and maybe you can relate to that. These feelings can take away our attachment to humanity and even cause us to lose hope. We simply cannot allow a person living with dementia to feel this way, day in and day out of their lives. It's up to us to make the difference because many times, they literally cannot find a handle to open a door. But we can. As their caregivers, we can encourage and cue their brains to route around roadblocks and help them use a different path. We can give voice and meaning to their communication that no longer makes sense. We can lead them to the door and help them step through into a life that is present and purposeful.

four

Know Their Needs

We force them to feel uncomfortable when we
meet our needs, instead of theirs.

Caring for a person with dementia is sometimes similar to caring for a baby; you have to know (or sometimes guess) their needs as a caregiver, just as you would a baby. Infants cannot verbally express their needs but that doesn't take away the fact those needs must be met for them to be happy and content and quit screaming their heads off!

anticipate needs

Someone suffering with dementia is in the same situation. Their ability to recognize and communicate needs becomes less and less the further progressed they become in the disease process. Even in early stages, though they may recognize a need, they don't always get it communicated clearly. This doesn't mean that we treat them like a baby; they are adults and deserve to be treated with the respect and regard they have earned throughout their lives. What it does mean is that we seek to anticipate their needs.

That sounds simple enough. But as you may have already discovered, this can be difficult with certain individuals. To be successful in this venture you must know the person you're caring for really well. You must get down to the nitty-gritty and ask for personal details that shed light on their inner soul. Whether you are caring for a family member or a resident in a senior living community, you need to find out who they are inside. If they can communicate well through a conversation, ask them:

"When you were a child, what did you dream about doing when you grew up?"

"If you could travel anywhere in the world right now, where would you go?"

"What do you love?"

"Name one person who has influenced you the most in your life."

If they can't answer, ask other family members or friends. These kinds of details give you insight into their personality and help you understand how to approach them when faced with the difficulty of interpreting needs. Knowing their past dreams, interests, hobbies and desires; whether they were from a large family or an only child; tells you a lot about their social interaction and makes it easier for us to identify circumstances that make them uncomfortable. Knowing that a person really loved nature and the sun on their face gives you a major clue to that inner, emotional need to get outdoors often. We have to help them fulfill these needs. You anticipate needs based on who they are as an individual but also from a basic understanding of bodily functions.

for example:

When dealing with the challenge of incontinence, if we could remind and direct the person to use the restroom every two hours, they would be less likely to have accidents, which eliminates the need to change briefs, pads or clothing as often. In the end, this saves time. Directing someone to the restroom can take a matter of seconds whereas having to help them change layers of clothing can take three times as long. We all generally need to use the bathroom after meals. But a person with dementia may feel this urge and not realize this feeling for what it actually is. Suddenly, they may start becoming anxious or agitated and really, all they need to do is take "a nature break" as one of my previous residents kindly put it. Think about how little kids will say they have a stomachache when what they really need to do is use the bathroom. Why not address the need before it occurs instead of waiting for a negative response? Schedule regular bathroom breaks. This makes total sense. By anticipating this need, we're simply cueing and beating the body to the punch line before it bursts. It's the same for all of our basic human needs whether we're hungry, in pain, sad, angry, or even excited. We take for granted that we retain the ability to recognize, interpret and act upon our physical feelings or reminders of these needs. Not so with a person living with dementia. Knowing and understanding this is a big deal because you can ward off 99% of what many caregivers deem "bad behavior" if you can address the probability of these needs before the outward symptoms are exhibited.

The Alzheimer's Association famously says, "behaviors are communication." How many of us get a little grouchy and short-tempered when we're in pain? If a dementia patient has other health concerns that are known to cause pain, we should be prepared to offer pain management whether they're able to pinpoint that as a problem or not, because given the situation, it is very likely they are experiencing pain. Pain is a hugely motivating factor for human beings. There will always be some sort of reaction to pain.

Take it a little further and realize that whatever routine a person has had throughout their lives has now become an actual need because it is hard wired in their brains. Maybe they had a cup of coffee in bed every morning at 6AM and nighttime snack at 9PM. Just because they don't remember this routine doesn't take away the importance of it to their body. Humans are very patterned individuals. Even a normal, healthy person can get irritable when they're thrown off track of their routine. Imagine what it must be like for someone who is confused and disorientated? We force them to feel uncomfortable when we meet our needs instead of theirs. The simplest way to define this dilemma may sound crude, but follow it and you can avoid difficult and challenging circumstances.

It's referred to in the industry as
"The Three P's: have they peed,
pooped or are they in pain?"

Taking care of these basic bodily functions is a big priority in good caregiving. You must know and anticipate their needs so that you can meet them.

five

Communicate Effectively

*We have to change our communication
approach because they cannot change the
disabled parts of their brain.*

A person battling dementia cannot communicate like you or I. The disease is killing their brain and body. Behaviors, anxiety and discontent are attempts to communicate an unmet need, often of which is not recognized by the person themselves. It becomes difficult for them to communicate because the disease is affecting the brain's ability to recognize and interpret stimuli. Some patients may actually hear you, but they can't process the sound. Their ability to take what they hear and categorize it into something that makes sense is suddenly gone. I had a resident tell me once, as we were passing a small group of staff in conversation:

> *"It sounds like they're talking
> through their nose."*

Judging from the blank looks that appear on the faces of persons with dementia at times, I imagine it sounds very much like we are speaking in a foreign language. If you've ever been in the company of people who were speaking in a language you couldn't understand, and you needed to understand them, it's a very isolating feeling. You may have heard of the "Virtual Dementia Tour"® created by P.K. Beville and promoted through Second Wind Dreams. It was created in attempt to help those who don't have dementia, understand what it feels like for someone living with dementia.

They have created a "window into their world" using an experimental kit where the participants put on goggles, gloves, and earphones; essentially impairing the senses and limiting their ability to interpret stimuli. They are then placed in an environment with further distractions and asked to perform specific tasks. I went through this experiment offered at a seminar I attended in 2011. At that point, I had been working with dementia for ten years and thought I had a pretty good understanding of what they dealt with. The *Virtual Dementia Tour®* opened my eyes. It deepened my level of empathy for those battling this horrible disease.

As caregivers, it is our job to help a person with dementia experience successful communication. Words begin holding less meaning, especially in latter stages. Verbal communication gets thrown on the back burner and instead, it's those non-verbal communication cues that come to the forefront. *How* you say it. *What* your body posture is signaling. Suddenly, the tone and pitch of your voice becomes more important than the words coming out of your mouth. The mind of dementia begins to think of language in a completely different way. It confuses words and sorts sentence structure in a pattern that doesn't make sense and the person with dementia can do nothing about this. Essentially, they begin speaking a different language. Yet it's a language common to every victim of this disease. In order for us to learn how to communicate with them, we have to learn how to speak like them. I have often said:

It's like learning a new language, and if you listen to them, they will teach you.

Just pay attention to how they are talking to you and begin to emulate their pattern. We have to change our approach and modify our usual means of communication because they cannot change the disabled parts of their brain. Obviously as the disease progresses it becomes harder for the person with dementia to function and communicate as we do. The following points can be applied in every level of the disease process. Keep in mind that these are communication tips, not necessarily general rules of thumb for handling the disease overall. But I guarantee, these tips will help you communicate better with your loved one.

Break it down

Use task segmentation. This means you don't list all the instructions at once. Give them one step at a time. You can express the final goal, but list each step separately and allow time for completion before moving on to the next step. A person battling mid-to-late stages of dementia needs a lot of cueing. But we want to give them the opportunity to function independently for as long as possible. Spell it out simply for them. On the next page is an example of how to break down the task of brushing your teeth.

Task Segmentation: Brushing Teeth

Step 1: Instruct, *"We are going to brush your teeth now."*
Step 2: Hand them their toothbrush as you say, *"Here's your toothbrush."*
Step 3: Hand them toothpaste as you say, *"Put some toothpaste on your toothbrush."*
Step 4: Verbally cue, *"Put the toothbrush in your mouth and brush your teeth."* Cue them physically with your hand if necessary.

Even in beginning stages, breaking instructions down into one step at a time tasks gives a person with dementia the ability to still do things on their own, instead of having everything done for them. It offers them a sense of dignity and treats them like the adult that they are, which we all deserve.

Slow down

Their life already feels like a merry-go-round because they are constantly trying to interpret stimuli. Don't add to the spin cycle. Literally slow down your actions, reactions and the way you speak. Create time and space. Don't rush.

Don't over stimulate.

We have all experienced what it's like to feel like you're in a fog and your brain is just not working. In these feelings, how much easier is it to navigate your own home with familiar and predictable stimuli rather than a crowded airport or noisy grocery store with all the sights, sounds and smells going on? It is important for the person with dementia to continue living and enjoying their life as they used to. But remember that *constant* stimulation can equal *negative* stimulation.

Reduce distraction

When attempting to communicate, keep the focus on one thing at a time. Turn off the radio and the TV unless you're actually listening or watching it. Don't expect a person with dementia to be able to follow you in conversation if five feet away, some-one else is having a very loud conversation of their own, or there are other distractions going on. Step away from distractions when trying to communicate.

Limit your word count

The less amount of words they have to take in, recognize and interpret into something that makes sense, the higher success rate you're going to have in being understood.

Say what you need to say
in the least amount of words possible.

Think back to watching the old cartoon, *Charlie Brown*. It's sort of like when an adult talks, all everyone hears is: *"Whah, Wa, Wah, Whah, Wah."* If you are speaking too fast or saying too much, it just sounds like an obnoxious noise in their ears and they have no idea what you are saying.

Watch your tone

I cannot stress the importance of this factor in effective communication even for those of us who don't have dementia! I can't tell you how many times my own husband has said, *"It's not what you said; it's how you said it."* Improper tone and voice inflection can cause a world of damage. You may be irritated with your loved one who is not doing something properly, but we must remember that they cannot help it.

Working in a secured care living environment, there are many times when a resident will attempt to get out a door. As staff, we know that it's a secure environment for their own safety. As a resident, all they know is that this isn't home or work or any place they recognize and therefore, this is not where they're supposed to be. In their mind, they have responsibilities that they are not fulfilling and this is upsetting to them. That is the mindset they're in. But rushing a resident who is trying to get out the door and yelling, *"Wait! Stop!"* Or *"Get back!"* only alarms them further. Instead, if you approach calmly, softly and most importantly with a friendly facial expression and tone of voice, you will be far more successful in getting them to listen to what you have to say and stop doing the "improper" action they are currently engaging in. Approach with a smile and say:

"Hi! There you are! I've been looking for you."

Roll into a conversation that builds a sense of camaraderie; a need for the two of you to be doing something together.

"Can you come help me with... (insert task)."

-or-

"Before we can leave, we have to... (insert task)."

Setting a friendly tone with your voice is the first step.

Check your body language

Similar to above, but of course the non-verbal side. You may be smiling, but is your posture demonstrating a friendly tone? Your body should express a relaxing atmosphere. Not rigid, hurried or stressed. A person with dementia is going to mirror your body language.

Use gestures

Rather than verbally over explaining something, use hand gestures to demonstrate what you're saying.

for example:

Let's imagine that you want them to get up out of the recliner in the living room and come to the kitchen for lunch. Get in front of them where they can clearly see you, make eye contact and say as you motion with your hands:

"Come with me. Let's go have lunch together."

Don't hover over them or go to their side and start physically pulling them up and out of their chair. You're invading their personal space and even if you have already told them that it's time for lunch, they may have forgotten and don't understand why you're suddenly tugging on them. Give them visual clues to go with the verbal request.

Respect their words

Do not write them off simply because they are confused, disorientated or don't know what they are doing. Even if you're trying to help and assist them in accomplishing a necessary task, if they tell you "*No*", you *must* respect this. If you disregard their words, not only are you taking away their rights and dignity, you're also completely devaluing any trust you've had or built with them. It doesn't matter who is wrong or who is right, all parties involved deserve to *feel* mutually respected. Our actions have to communicate that.

As long as they are not putting themselves or someone else in danger, respect what they are telling you. When what they say is contrary to your goal, first of all, reassess the necessity of your goal. Second, rethink your approach. Were you too demanding or authoritative? Did you approach too rapidly and put them on the defensive? Can you word your task in a different manner that makes more sense to them? This also relates to a previous point about understanding who the person is and knowing their needs. Let's say that your loved one with dementia needs assistance with bathing and dressing. In years prior, they've always taken a bath before bed. But maybe it's easier for us to take care of this task in the morning. How accepting do you think they're going to be when we wake them up and tell them to get up and out of bed because it's time for a bath? More than likely, you'll end up with an unpleasant confrontation. When we know this information, it is much easier to approach them in a manner that respects their wishes. Further, if they don't actually need full assistance with personal care, don't insist upon being there. Get them set up, check in on them and allow them some personal pride and independence. No one likes to be treated as though they are incompetent.

six

Offer Acceptance

Join them where they are.

, I have said that in dementia care, we simply join them where they are. We need to be the lifeline that reconnects them to meaningful living. In the midst of the chaos and confusion of their mind, a hug takes all the noise away; a look of acknowledgement is all that is needed to calm the soul; a kiss on the cheek and an *"I love you"* can melt anger into tears of relief because then, you are a person who is known and understood. A person with dementia wants that personal connection. They constantly feel lost, stuck and alone. They need to feel connected. The further progressed they get in the disease process the harder it is for them to feel that way. They need a lot of help to simply recognize their own feelings. It takes that individual approach, from someone who knows and understands them. As caregivers, something in our approach has to tell them:

I know you. We know each other.
You are important to me.

In this approach, we are offering emotional safety. Years ago, I had one particular resident that often wandered the building looking for her daughter, mother, or sister. When she couldn't find them, she would eventually become so distraught that her sobbing was practically inconsolable. In her mind, since she couldn't find them, something terrible must have happened to them and as she often said, after her unsuccessful searching:

"They must be dead."

As a caregiver in a senior living setting, we can never take the place of family. But if we can help meet the emotional need for intimacy and love, these distraught feelings do not surface as frequently. In a community setting, when a person is trying to leave the building constantly (which is their current living situation), I believe this action tells us that some emotional need is not being fulfilled. Persons with dementia function largely off of their emotions. What can we do, right now, in their moment of distress and confusion to meet this need for love and acceptance and offer them a sense of value and connection? I imagine if they could express these feelings of loneliness, it might sounds like this...

Just call my name and take my hand and say nothing else, but accept me. Because I cannot explain what I feel. My words don't make sense and your words are a language I no longer understand. But your eyes, they know me. They tell me everything is ok, and at least for now, I am not alone.

No one wants to feel emotionally deserted. We need to feel the push and pull of interaction. For all the elders I've known battling dementia, they teach me the importance of every interaction. Nothing is in vain. Inside my head, I feel like they are saying:

Every moment matters because the next time I see you, I may not know who you are. But you are life to me right now. You are real. You are here, and I am so scared of what is to come. So be with me now, for I don't know what the next moment may bring.

This is what I feel they teach me, and such wisdom they have, for they recognize there is no time to make it look pretty. No time for appearances. It is raw openness and honesty and there is such purity there. They may not know your name but they know if you've invested in them. You must ask yourself when you witness someone "failing to thrive" which is an industry term for someone who has basically given up on living; is it because this is what they want? Are they ready to be done? Or have we failed to help them still feel of value to live? We must offer them arms of acceptance and join them where THEY are.

In the short time I've been doing this, I see the payback. I experience the love and friendship those with dementia share with me. I see the family member eight years later who says, *"I remember you!"* And I can reply, *"Oh! What a difference your loved one made in my life,"* and mean it. Those connections are never lost. They continue to live on. As passe' as that may sound, it reverberates to my core and I know, this much is true. Sharing my life with these beautiful and amazing people, who also happen to have dementia, has made me a softer, calmer and more peaceful person. Their spirit continues to live, through each breath I take.

seven

Renew a Sense of Control

*Invite them to make choices in their life
because it is still, their life.*

How would you feel if you had everything taken away from you? Your job, your home, your car, your family, your social life, your money, your independence and then on top of that, to slowly watch it happen? This is what happens to a person experiencing Alzheimer's disease. Because of this, they often feel an extreme sense of loss. I had a resident tell me once:

> *"You might as well put me in an empty house and burn it down."*

When I asked why, he replied with:

> *"Well, I can't be with my family, so what's the point?"*

This tearing away from their family is a very painful wound. We don't want to focus on their loss; but we do want to recognize *what* they've lost so we can attempt to fill this void with opportunities for them to feel empowered. We must help them express their individual opinions and make their own decisions.

I see it happen quite often: once a person is diagnosed with dementia, the caregiver automatically goes into defense mode. It's a natural "fight or flight" response. They feel the need to defend against this disease that's now changing both their life and that of their loved one. A caregiver often feels like they are left all alone to make these decisions about the future. But there are still so many areas where the person diagnosed with the disease can still function very well. Maybe it's easier for you to decide what they're wearing, eating or doing and when they're doing all of those things. But you're inhibiting their personal choices (and rights) by not allowing them to be a part of the process. Ask them for their opinion. Allow them the opportunity to think for themselves:

Where would you like to eat dinner?

What kind of food sounds good?

Where should I hang this picture?

Allowing them control over a decision, or the ability to affect an outcome is hugely gratifying.

———————————

By allowing them a sense of control,
you are giving their words and therefore
their life as an individual, value and purpose.

———————————

Ask them for opinions about real things too, not just the lighthearted, daily parts of living, though there's nothing wrong with that. Go ahead and talk about religion and politics, not to share your views, but to listen to theirs.

encourage individuality

How important is it for you to feel like you're alive in the present world? For those of us not battling dementia, that's a feeling we easily take for granted. We all have times where we want to turn off our brain and think about mindless things or talk about something easy like the weather. But sometimes we want to feel attached to the more important areas of life too. So don't forget how important that may be to someone who is literally losing their life.

In later stages of the disease, caring for the person with dementia becomes more centered around direct care of their physical needs: eating, using the bathroom, sleep, or medication. But often in the midst of completing these tasks, the goal becomes centered around making things easier on the caregiver. This frequently happens in residential care communities where individual staff members are responsible for completing many tasks all in a day's work. But we are in the business of caring for people and we can't forget this. Our job should not be built around what's easier for us, but what fits the individual needs of the resident. We need to reverse the direction and keep the focus on the person we are caring for.

Encouraging independence
increases function.

This brings about less dependence on the caregiver and makes the job *easier*. Aiding in their independence, or at least encouraging those feelings, makes a person battling dementia happier. And when they are happy, things move smoother.

Caregivers should practice an intentional approach that lends to renewing a sense of control in the mind of the person with dementia. I touched on a little of this in the earlier section about communication and respecting their words. It's easy to get too focused on the task we're trying to accomplish and forget that they deserve a say in what's happening. So again, don't tell them what to do. Instead, gently cue them to action in such a respectful manner that they feel like they had a say in the matter.

Which of the following would you prefer to hear?

> *"Sit down, (insert your name).*
> *Here. Sit down in this chair."*
>
> - or -
>
> *"Here, (insert name). This seat is for you.*
> *I saved it just for you."*

There is a difference between a command and an invitation. And it gives a sense of control simply by how you worded it. Offer them an invitation to engage in making choices in their life because it is still, *their* life. On the following page, I have included the Best Friends (TM) Dementia Bill of Rights from The Best Friends (TM) Approach to Dementia Care, Second Edition (2015), by Virginia Bell and David Troxel. © Health Professions Press, Incorporated. Virginia and David have done an amazing job advocating for persons with dementia and developing techniques for care that are solely focused around the client, not the caregiver. I believe that if you truly understand and implement these rights in your caregiving practice, you will empower a sense of control AND enable your ability for better care. Again, we force those with dementia to feel uncomfortable when we meet our needs, instead of theirs.

DEMENTIA BILL OF RIGHTS

- To be informed of one's diagnosis
- To have appropriate, ongoing medical care
- To be treated as an adult, listened to, and afforded respect for one's feelings and point of view
- To be with individuals who know one's life story, including cultural and spiritual traditions
- To experience meaningful engagement throughout the day
- To live in a safe and stimulating environment
- To be outdoors on a regular basis
- To be free from psychotropic medications whenever possible
- To have welcomed physical contact, including hugging, caressing and hand-holding
- To be an advocate for oneself and for others
- To be a part of a local, global or online community
- To have care partners well trained in dementia care

Dementia Bill of Rights
www.healthpropress.com
Reprinted by permission

eight

Don't Argue

*The truth is, their brain is lying to them.
And there's nothing in the world that we
can say or do to change that fact.*

You will never win an argument with a person with dementia. Logic and reason are no longer qualities that their compromised brain retains. This is especially hard for us to believe when we're dealing with someone in the early stages of memory loss, because they seem still "with it". Their conversation skills are still largely intact and we think this means that we can share a logical conversation with them. But the truth is, their brain is lying to them and there's nothing in the world that we can say or do to change that fact. Whatever is "real" in their mind, is very real. This is the biggest piece of advice I share with family members.

As long as what they believe is not hurting themselves or someone else, roll with it.

Believe it right along with them. It's important that we validate their feelings, regardless of the current state of their reality. If you can't successfully learn to do this, you are going to have a very hard time caring for your loved one. They are *always* right. In the grand scheme of things, is it worth arguing about whether they just finished one bowl of ice cream, and therefore they can't have another? Or whether they just saw Aunt Mary from California yesterday, when really she's been gone for ten years? If you end up in a situation where they are angry with you, back off. Respect their personal space and give them room to breathe. Reverse the roles and imagine that you are the angry one. What type of reaction or resolution would you want? This mental switch is a good problem solving technique. It's just like the old saying: *"put yourself in their shoes."* When you feel powerless, someone telling you how to feel or what to do only intensifies that feeling. As a caregiver, it's our job to not make the situation worse by pointing out error. In dementia care when a person is upset and acting out in ways we find irrational and unreasonable, the last thing you should do is to try and reason with them. You don't argue but instead, creatively find tactics to both validate them and redirect their thought process. You don't try to orientate them to the current reality, but rather communicate to them that you are on "their side" and they are safe. You can read more in depth about this technique by researching *"validation therapy"*. It's another very common industry practice in dementia care.

In late stages of the disease, although they may not recognize where they are or who they may be surrounded by, you communicate to them with your presence and tone of voice that you know them and everything is going to be ok. Essentially you are orientating them to you and the safety you offer.

That's why it's important to build a relationship of trust with those with dementia, so that you *can* reassure them in the midst of an emotionally tense situation. We must find ways to redirect their brain off the topic that is upsetting them and subsequently help de-escalate their anxiety and emotions.

nine

Redirection and Distraction

*Turn the emphasis away from
the negative factor.*

Rather than argue, it is much better to redirect the energy. You distract their attention and focus it on something else. Turn the emphasis away from the negative factor and find a common factor that you know will bring about a positive reaction from the individual. Try using some of the following techniques:

❖ Use of touch (slowly and gently start rubbing their back; unless they are angry, in which case they usually need their personal space respected). In cases of exhibited anxiety, the use of touch can be very comforting.

❖ Food (this is easy, immediate and highly effective).

❖ Animals (the gentle and quiet companionship of an animal is instantly soothing, IF they like animals).

❖ Action or task (give them something to do; put them in a "helping" role).

❖ Offer to turn on some of their favorite music, or movie/TV show.

❖ Look at personal items/or photos. Make your interaction a personal one by reflecting on items that you know they enjoy or have sentimental value to them. Such as: pictures; their hand-made quilt; a typewriter they used daily; antique dishes; etc.

You'll notice many of these call upon the senses. These forms of stimuli are areas of non-verbal communication. Our senses use a different area of the brain than verbal communication does. Prompting the person's thought process away from the logic and reason side of the brain can have the ultimate success of distraction. Mention the sunshine (or the rain) outside; or the smell of dinner cooking; or the sound of someone laughing followed by: *"Let's go have a look. It sounds like something is going on!"* Often in this field, caregivers use a technique called *therapeutic lying*.

Therapeutic lying is when you tell a little white lie for the purpose of protecting the emotional well-being of a person battling dementia.

It's important to differentiate here: that you do not lie to protect yourself from dealing with their emotions, but to protect them and their feelings. You do have to be careful how you implement this technique because no matter what stage of the disease you're dealing with, a person with dementia can sometimes interpret if you're flat out lying to them. So, it's really more like bending the truth a little. Again, remember that it's ultimately about validating their reality and joining them in it.

for example:

Let's say your loved one, or a new resident at a care community, is determined to get in their car and go somewhere, but they haven't been able to drive in years (or obviously can't now). Here is what you can say to them:

> *"Your car is not here. Your son/daughter/*
> *brother (fill-in-the-blank) had to borrow it*
> *for an appointment. They will call you*
> *when they're through."*

Maybe they want to take a bus or call a taxi (I've had this happen)... to which I replied:

> *"The bus is through running for the day. No*
> *more stops today. We'll catch it tomorrow."*

-or maybe-

> *"Your family made arrangements for you to stay for the evening. We're getting dinner ready for you; you have a very nice apartment for the night; and they'll call you in the morning."*

Notice, you're not telling them they get to leave tomorrow but you are redirecting (or distracting) them from thinking about leaving, *right now*. You can bend the truth a little where you need to (the family borrowed the car) and then redirect the conversation elsewhere by making the situation sound temporary and talking about something else (like dinner, or the next non-threatening thing on the agenda).

Here's another good example. I was in the middle of an art therapy class when I noticed a resident who was sitting alone and crying, silently. I approached her softly and slowly in an attempt to comfort her:

> *"Why are you crying?"* I ask.
> In between a very jumbled collection of words, I understood she was trying to say:
> *"Where are my children? I need to get to them, now! Where are they?"*
> *"Oh Gerry. It's OK."* I try to reassure her.
> *"No! It's not!"* She bursts out.
> *"But they're safe."* I say.

"How? How do you know that?"
She asks.
I search my brain quickly, thinking for a
response: *"They're at school. It's the middle of
the day and they're at school with their teachers.
Trust me. Everything is ok."*

It took a few more minutes of reassurance but the
tears finally stopped and she looked at me and
said,

"Thank you. You're very kind."

I probably would not have been successful in redirecting and comforting her if I hadn't previously
built a relationship with her and earned her trust.
This is a very important factor in working with dementia. You must establish a foundation of trust
between yourself and the individual. You validate
and earn trust. In this particular instance, some part
of her recognized that feeling of trust as she looked
into my eyes during my attempts to calmly reassure her that her children were safe and all was
well. She is always worried about where her family
is. This is a common occurrence, especially in mid-
to-late stages of the disease as the brain deteriorates
and they lose orientation to time and place. They
revert back to much earlier years of their life when

for most women, their main daily concern was caring for their children and family. We need to surround them with love and nurture them with support.

ten

Laugh It Off

*Laughter lightens the emotional mood and
instantly decreases the stress of any situation.*

When all else fails, let go and laugh. We're all familiar with the old saying, *"Laughter is the best medicine."* I'll add to that with: *"and it is healing to the soul."* People with dementia love to laugh! Who doesn't like to laugh? It lightens the emotional mood and instantly decreases the stress of any situation.

Laughter releases "happy" endorphins in the brain. It also builds an instant sense of camaraderie, community and solidarity. Laughter encourages a positive attitude and a positive approach does wonders as you seek answers for negative behaviors.

You want a positive response?
You must give a positive address.

Have some fun! Role-play some ridiculous idea or engagement! This is where joining their reality literally can mean playing along with the story! Think of it as though you are creatively exploring together and exploring can be both exciting and invigorating! One of my favorite party games is "Catch Phrase". It's the modern form of charades. Engaging in some sort of silliness gets everyone on a more lighthearted page.

You can research all the positive effects laughter can have on the body. But my favorite effect of this technique is that rather than finding yourself in a negative situation with your loved one, you end up laughing together. The person with dementia may not remember that exact occasion tomorrow, but the more you laugh with them, the more often you find it easier to elicit a positive response from them. You both get used to the pattern of smiling together and begin to unconsciously form a habit of happiness in each other's company. Create happiness and laugh with wild, reckless abandon!

eleven

Remain Calm

You absolutely, cannot take anything personally.
Calmness gives the illusion of control
and offers a sense of security.

I know that dealing with this disease can be frustrating. But the moment you express frustration, you put the person with dementia on edge, heightening anxiety and often triggering negative responses. There have been many times when I have been caught in a difficult situation with a resident, often experiencing the brunt of their anger. It is with great patience that I remind myself: their reality may not make sense to me, but it's *very* real to them and I must maintain a calm composure.

You absolutely, cannot take
anything personally.

It is not their fault. It is not them speaking or acting; it is the disease. They may believe that their mother is waiting for them to come home, and they are about to either be in big trouble or worry their poor mother to death! This anxiety is very real and is causing the response you are now witnessing. I've said this repeatedly: *join them where they are.* If you are anxious and frustrated, they will begin to exhibit similar feelings and responses. They are extremely sensitive to the mood and energy surrounding them. To remain calm, you must let go of your own feelings and partner with them in validating their feelings.

allow space for erratic behavior

The last thing you want to do is make a person with dementia feel like a crazy person. Because they already feel this way! The better you make them feel, the calmer they become. Allow time and space in your interactions. They need this extra space to process what's happening around them.

for example

Think back to a time when you were in the middle of an argument with someone and the two of you were going back and forth over an issue. Did it ever help the situation to call the other person "crazy" or "wrong"? In my experience, that's just like poking a sleeping bear. We all have a right to our feelings. Whether they are justified or not is another matter. But if we recognize that dementia robs the individual of the ability to process things in a rational manner, it's easier for us to not take things personally and allow space for their reactions or behaviors that make no sense.

the mirror effect

People living with dementia often mirror the mood of their surrounding environment. This is why it is so important for you to remain calm because your composure projects into them and it assures them that although things may feel chaotic, everything is actually just fine. It is giving the illusion that everything is under control and reinforcing the fact that they are safe.

Stop and take a deep breath before you respond. It's that little trick of creating time and space; leaving dead air so calmness can appear.

twelve

Be Consistent

*Consistency breeds familiarity and
familiarity brings comfort.*

When a person is already confused, it's very difficult to be surrounded by faces you don't recognize. Large groups can be very overwhelming. Limiting group size in residential activities and even family events can be helpful. Also keep in mind, that being cared for in a very personal way by someone who appears to be a stranger can trigger an immediate feeling of fear. Many residential care communities are recognizing this fact and are subsequently scheduling their staffing to fit a more consistent pattern; where the same individuals work the exact same shift throughout the week. This lends to decreasing the stranger syndrome because some area of the brain and body is now familiar with the faces and routine of this pattern. It's important to change the routine of a person with dementia as little as possible. As the disease progresses, there will be many things that become unsafe to remain a part of a daily routine. But we can make modifications to keep their daily routine in action. Although we may not always be aware of it, we are very patterned individuals. We find comfort in routine. Remaining in a familiar environment offers those with dementia a genuine sense of security. We must offer comfort and security through our caregiving.

If and when you arrive at a point of recognizing that your loved one needs more care than you can continue to give, it may be time for them to move into a senior healthcare environment. Most families faced with this dilemma often wait much longer than they should to make this decision. It's best to consider this move while your loved one retains some ability to become orientated to their surroundings. I personally believe that if a person with dementia has the opportunity to transition their living environment in earlier stages of the disease, they can adjust and relate to their surroundings better. It has the chance of becoming a familiar place at a quicker rate. Otherwise, it can be very scary because they don't recognize anything and this heightens feelings of confusion.

thirteen

Using Therapeutic Outlets

Time after time it's become evident to me that the creative and artistic outlets seem to transcend the disease within the brain.

As part of recreational and therapeutic programming in senior living communities, we implement art, music, horticultural, spiritual, pet therapy, and many other forms of therapy and stimulation. Not only does this offer enrichment to daily living, it provides a non-verbal medium where a person with dementia can communicate their feelings and emotions in an unencumbered state. Dementia puts roadblocks in the paths of communication. Various therapy techniques can assist in routing around these roadblocks.

The quality of programming provided in dementia care matters. We need to continue stimulating the mind and exercise areas of the brain that are still active in order to keep these areas maintained and accessible for longer periods of time. The brain learns to compensate for the damaged areas and this often results in a "new" learned ability in another area of function. That's why it's not uncommon for a person with dementia to suddenly learn new talents or do something they've never done before. There are studies and ongoing research popping up in this area all the time. A past study "Brain reserve hypothesis in dementia" published in *Journal of Alzheimer's Disease* (2007) notates the brain actually reserves cognitive function based on factors such as education, level of work difficulty and degree of social interaction. It makes the point that the brain leans on these reserves and functional abilities when it begins to become compromised. Further findings by Randy Buckner in "Memory and executive function in aging and Alzheimer's disease," discovered that Alzheimer's disease "preferentially affects the medial temporal lobe and this disruption leads directly to memory impairment." Studied images of a brain affected by Alzheimer's in this study show increased activity in certain areas of the brain, and that this "extra recruitment may [have been] reflecting a form of compensation." What this means is: when one part of the brain dies, the parts that are still living sort of kick into high gear to pick up the slack.

Working in the field of recreational therapy, I have had many opportunities to experiment with implementing various types of creative and therapeutic outlets for persons with dementia. The following pages share some personal stories surrounding these experiences.

Poetry Corner

Years ago, when I first started working in dementia care, I would periodically gather a small group of residents and hold an impromptu Poetry Corner. After selecting a specific poem, we'd read it together, discuss its meaning and then proceed to write our own poem on the subject. It became a very meaningful time as we shared our feelings, memories and emotions. In one particular group we read the following poem by William Butler Yeats:

A Memory of Youth

The moments passed as at a play;
I had the wisdom love brings forth;
I had my share of mother wit,
And yet for all that I could say,
And though I had her praise for it,
A cloud blown from the cutthroat North
Suddenly hid Love's moon away.
Believing every word I said,
I praised her body and her mind
Till pride had made her eyes grow bright,
And pleasure made her cheeks grow red,
And vanity her foot fall light,
Yet we, for all that praise, could find
Nothing but darkness overhead.
We sat silent as a stone,
We knew, though she'd not said a word,
That even the best of love must die,
And had been savagely undone
Were it not the Love upon the cry
Of a most ridiculous little bird
Tore from the clouds his marvelous moon.

Although crowds gathered one
If she but showed her face,
And even old men's eyes grew dim,
This hand alone,
Like some last courtier
At a gypsy camping place
Babbling of fallen majesty,
Records what gone.
These lineaments,
A heart that laughter has made sweet,
These, these remain,
But I record what's gone.
A crowd will gather,
And not know it walks the very street
Whereon a thing once walked
That seemed a burning cloud.

This poem spurred a conversation about lost love. I asked them if they thought there was a timeline for love. We discussed what it felt like to be in love; how when you have it, you feel like you're on top of the world; you feel as though you've gained a sense of newfound knowledge! Yet suddenly, something can happen and it disappears; or something can take it away, like death. Many of these seniors were living without spouses now. I believe they identified with this poem by Yeats. All the sweet-talking in the world didn't keep their love from dying; it doesn't keep Yeats from these feelings of emptiness and loneliness as people pass him by, having no idea of the burning intensity of love once there. We talked about love for quite awhile, as I took notes. Here is the poem we created together in 2005, on the subject of young love.

Young Love

Young love, fluttering like a butterfly
Vivid dreams, dancing in your head.
The feeling of cold, clammy skin
Hoping the feeling would fade away
As we become more near and dear.
With familiarity comes a calm
At last, just like the song.
Closer we become
Through the good, the bad, the ugly
And all of life's uncertainty.
Just like the first time
Of a nervous butterfly's flight
We have made it through,
All the happenings in this life.
Love is our gift from God
That we will always have,
No timeline can that rob away
We have it through each day.

In yet another session, we read a poem about discovering hobbies and how rewarding it was to spend time doing the things you love. When I asked them to talk about their hobbies, it was interesting to see how many hobbies were related to things they did throughout the day, around the house, or for their occupations. I did this session several times throughout the years. *Reminiscing In Hobbies* is a poem that was created in 2003. I can still see the faces of the individuals in this poem, as they smiled and shared their life stories with me.

Reminiscing in Hobbies

The time of day is 2 o'clock
It's ready to start the cooking
Oh how much there was to do
But out the window Fannie keeps looking.

Frank was practicing his golf swing
To Colorado he was headed for a match
There was much, much practicing to do
Aiming the ball, hoping the hole would catch.

In town Charlotte is at the cosmetic shop
Lucky she is, to work in a hobby she enjoys,
The many people she gets to meet and help
Choose the many colors of makeup,
    as their toys.

Down at the water hole, Mary is a lookin'
For the many fish that she can hook,
Catching fish was what she loved
Down by her country crook.

Flowers were Hedy's first love
Roses were here favorite bloom
The many colors surrounding her
Were always enough to cut the darkest gloom.

At the end of the day
We all head to town
To listen to Bob and his accordion
Tearing the house down!

Of course, we all have hobbies. But as they shared this part of themselves, I witnessed a joy in their eyes that took them out of that moment and into a place beyond. And that's exactly what hobbies are for: a reprieve from what we feel are obligations; a break from the normalcy of life, so to speak.

Pet therapy

The use of animals as a therapy tool can be a very nurturing experience for someone battling dementia. I remember one particular lady who was in the mid-to-late stages of Alzheimer's. Her body was still very physically healthy, but the disease was robbing her brain's ability to sort words and speech and therefore it was becoming difficult to understand much of anything she said or did. She was no longer orientated to objects and their proper use on a regular basis. You could barely understand her when she tried to talk. It was often jumbled words that made no sense and sometimes, it wasn't even words at all. But she could still walk and spent much of her day walking around, alone. She was a little bit of a loner. One day, I was around the corner from her in a hallway, and I could hear her talking to our community dog. It stopped me dead in my tracks because what I heard were actual words, in sentences that made complete sense!

"Hello doggie. You're so pretty! Yes, you are!
How are you doing today?"

As I rounded the corner to face her, she looked up at me and then said to the dog:

"Come on, let's go to Daddy."

Now, I'm not daddy, so she mixed up the words "Daddy" and "Mommy" but her speech was clear as a bell! For a woman who ordinarily made no sense at all in her speech, it made my soul jump with joy at this little personal conversation between her and the dog. The interaction with the dog returned her ability to clearly and concisely communicate. This is why we implement various forms of therapy into daily living and exactly why I vouch for therapies that utilize non-verbal medium that call upon our senses. Animals have the ability to communicate non-verbally and this speaks to the person with dementia in a way that makes them feel understood and accepted.

Art Therapy

I had another 90-year old lady in the early stages of dementia, who struggled to see because of macular degeneration. She had been a rural schoolteacher and loved to talk about those days. Remembering that period was reminding her of a time in life when she felt important and needed. It's so common for seniors to lose a portion of their self-esteem after moving to a senior living community, because suddenly they are no longer necessary in meeting the needs of others. Now other people are meeting their needs. One day, I was able to convince her to come to our art class. Throughout the session, she continually verbalized her frustration with her lack of ability to see what she was doing. But we kept reassuring her that she was doing a great job. She started coming every week and in the end, had a piece selected for the annual *Memories in the Making*® Art Auction with our local Alzheimer's Association. The pride and gratification of personally creating something that was recognized by others as important was a much needed gift to her.

Time after time it has become evident to me how these non-verbal and creative communication outlets seem to transcend the disease within the brain. We know through many educational and scientific sources that in reality, the creative areas of the brain are the last to be affected by the disease progression. But when you experience this transcendence in a personal moment with one of these patients, it's like watching a miracle unfold right in front of your eyes.

Music Therapy

I am also a musician, a pianist and vocalist, and I implement the use of music as therapy into daily programming as much a possible. It breaks down so many barriers. Countless times, as I've been playing and singing familiar tunes from their era of music, I've had residents who normally don't speak chime in singing with me the entire lyrics of a song. They don't know their own name, but they can sing "Oh Susanna" in a voice that belies any indication of a brain disorder.

There's a lot of developing research in the area of dementia and how exercising new skills can encourage brain function. I look forward to a future where living with dementia feels less like a death sentence and more like a new way of looking at life, with appreciation for every, single moment. I certainly feel, in my years of observing residents living in senior living communities that many of them feel undervalued and under appreciated. But caregivers can change that. It is my personal goal to empower those in this profession with a sense of love and communal bond with their clients and to encourage families to find creative ways to interact and engage with their loved ones. I truly believe it makes a huge difference.

I want to close this chapter with a poem entitled "Crabby Old Woman", author unknown. The internet lore surrounding this poem tells the story of a hospital in Scotland, where upon cleaning a room, staff ran across this poem scribbled on a piece of paper.

Crabby Old Woman

What do you see, what do you see?
What are you thinking, when you look at me -
A crabby old woman, not very wise,
Uncertain of habit, with far-away eyes,
Who dribbles her food and makes no reply

When you say in a loud voice,
"I do wish you'd try."
Who seems not to notice the things that you do
And forever is loosing a stocking or shoe.
Who, unresisting or not; lets you do as you will
With bathing and feeding the long day is full.
Is that what you're thinking?
Is that what you see?
Then open your eyes nurse,
You're looking at me.
I'll tell you who I am as I sit here so still,
As I rise at your bidding, as I eat at your will.
I'm a small child of ten with a father and mother,
Brothers and sisters, who loved one another.
A young girl of sixteen with wings on her feet,
Dreaming that soon now a lover she'll meet.
A bride soon at twenty - my heart gives a leap,
Remembering the vows that I promised to keep.
As twenty-five now I have young of my own
Who need me to build a secure happy home;
A woman of thirty, my young now grow fast,
Bound to each other with ties that should last;
At forty, my young sons have grown and are gone,
But my man is beside me to see I don't mourn;
At fifty once more babies play around my knee,
Again we know children, my loved one and me.
Dark days are upon me, my husband is dead,
I look at the future, I shudder with dread,
For my young are all rearing young of their own.

And I think of the years and the love that I've known;
I'm an old woman now and nature is cruel -
Tis her jest to make old age look like a fool.
There is now a stone where I once had a heart,
But inside this old carcass, a young girl still   dwells,
And now and again my battered heart swells,
I remember the joy, I remember the pain,
And I'm loving and living life over again.
I think of the years all too few - gone too fast.
And accept the stark fact that nothing can last.
So open your eyes, nurse, open and see,
Not a crabby old woman, look closer -
See Me.

fourteen

Give Love

Love initiates an intimacy that unites us all.
And then, we are no longer alone on this journey.

I lost two grandfathers with dementia. One was taken by a form of lung cancer, which induced dementia. And the other, passed from Alzheimer's disease slowly taking his body, one living cell at a time. It's a humbling experience to live day in and day out with people experiencing this disease. I saw firsthand the dedication it took on my grandmother's part, to give my grandfather the care he needed toward the end of his life. And she did it with great dignity. Love can cross boundaries that science cannot explain. Love gives you, the caregiver, the energy to continue when you feel as though you have nothing left to give. I am continually amazed by the strength, power and love I witness in my life. These truths have made a large impact on the woman I am today.

What a joy to honor the life and
energy that continually moves
inside each of us. There is no end.
The breath simply reinvents
itself to new purpose.

This is why I do this. To build bridges over what feels like a meaningless void. I can sink in and get lost in my own life sometimes. But I am sweetly reminded that I am needed; I am important; and I am loved. These reminders are what keep us living. I encourage you to move forward into a relationship with your loved one that is full of love. Give yourself grace to do this, because you *can* do this. Be kind to yourself. Give yourself a break when you need it. Walk away. No matter what has happened before today, you are now armed with a new knowledge. A warm embrace can melt everything away and words are no longer needed. A soft caress tells us that no matter how crazy we feel, we are loved. It initiates an intimacy that unites us, and we are no longer alone on this journey. I sincerely hope that your next step may be one of peace and love.

THANK YOU

Thank you my dear friends: Mary Nelson, Hedy, Bob, Frank, Charlotte, Leota, Stanley, Vincent, Lewanda, Martin, William, Tommy, Adelaide, Gladys, Helen & Bob Sterling, Betty, Dorothy, Martha Wainright, Melissa Hampton, Ray Hamm, Henry, Frances, Leila, Carol, Jeanette, Geraldine, Jean Powell, Patty Dunkin, Jack Swafford, Jim, Jan, Mildred, Ruth, Betty, Lois, Al & Verna, Nellie, Sigrid, Marilyn, Mary K, Maxine, Evanelle, Kay, Aileen, Ann & Ellis, Velma, Marcia, Tom, Dorla, Faye, Juanita, Margaret... and all the rest of those faces I see, yet whose names I cannot remember.

Thank you for the wisdom you shared.

NOTES

Callone, Patricia. Vasiloff, Barbara. Kudlacek, Connie. Manternach, Janaan. Brumback, Roger. *Alzheimer's Disease: The Dignity Within.* Demos Medical Publishing, 2006.

McLeod, Beth Witrogen. *And Thou Shalt Honor: The Caregiver's Companion.* Wiland-Bell Productions, 2002.

Arenella, Cheryl. "Alzheimer's Disease (and other Brain Diseases) and Hospice Care," *American Hospice Foundation.* 2007. Accessed via web May, 2013.

Fratiglioni, Laura, and Hui-Xin Wang. "Brain reserve hypothesis in dementia." *Journal of Alzheimer's disease* 12.1 (2007): 11-22.

Buckner, Randy L. "Memory and executive function in aging and AD: multiple factors that cause decline and reserve factors that compensate." *Neuron* 44.1 (2004): 195-208.

Alzheimer's Association. Professional advice and resources for families and caregivers living and working with this disease. www.alz.org

National Center for Creative Aging.
Dedicated to fostering an understanding of the vital relationship between creative expression and healthy aging. www.creativeaging.org

Second Wind Dreams. A patented sensory tool to help you empathize with those who have dementia. "Virtual Dementia Tour."® www.secondwind.org

University of Kansas Alzheimer's Disease Center. A National Institute of Aging designated research and disease center. www.kualzheimer.org

National Council of Certified Dementia Practition-ers. Promotes standards of excellence in dementia care and Alzheimer's disease education. www.nccdp.org

Alzheimer's Foundation of America.
Assures quality of care and excellence in service to individuals with Alzheimer's disease, and to their caregivers and families. www.alzfdn.org

RECOMMENDED READING

Bell, Virginia and Troxel, David. *A Dignified Life: The Best Friends Approach to Alzheimer's Care*. Health Communications, Inc. Rev. Exp. edition, 2012.

Brackey, Jolene. *Creating Moments of Joy*. Jolene Brackey, 2007.

McLeod, Beth Witrogen. *Caregiving: The Spiritual Journey of Love, Loss and Renewal*. Wiley, 2000.

Shouse, Deborah. *Love in the Land of Dementia*. Central Recovery Press, 2013.

Geonova, Lisa. *Still Alice*. Gallery Books, 2009.

Greenblat, Cathy. *Love, Loss and Laughter: Seeing Alzheimer's Differently*. Globe Pequot Press, 2012.

Coste, Joanne Koenig. *Learning to Speak Alzheimer's*. Mariner Books, 2004.

DeBiaggio, Thomas. *Losing My Mind*. The Free Press of Simon & Schuster Inc, 2002.